This Fucking Planner Belongs To:

TIME TO GET
THIS SHIT
STARTED

What is this badass planner going to do for you?

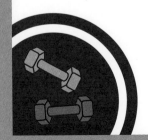

What's been stopping you from rocking this exercise shit before?

What are your long-term fitness goals?

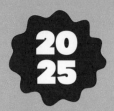 AT A GLANCE

JANUARY 2025

S	M	T	W	T	F	S
			1	2	3	4
5	6	7	8	9	10	11
12	13	14	15	16	17	18
19	20	21	22	23	24	25
26	27	28	29	30	31	

FEBRUARY 2025

S	M	T	W	T	F	S
						1
2	3	4	5	6	7	8
9	10	11	12	13	14	15
16	17	18	19	20	21	22
23	24	25	26	27	28	

MARCH 2025

S	M	T	W	T	F	S
						1
2	3	4	5	6	7	8
9	10	11	12	13	14	15
16	17	18	19	20	21	22
$23/30$	$24/31$	25	26	27	28	29

APRIL 2025

S	M	T	W	T	F	S
		1	2	3	4	5
6	7	8	9	10	11	12
13	14	15	16	17	18	19
20	21	22	23	24	25	26
27	28	29	30			

MAY 2025

S	M	T	W	T	F	S
				1	2	3
4	5	6	7	8	9	10
11	12	13	14	15	16	17
18	19	20	21	22	23	24
25	26	27	28	29	30	31

JUNE 2025

S	M	T	W	T	F	S
1	2	3	4	5	6	7
8	9	10	11	12	13	14
15	16	17	18	19	20	21
22	23	24	25	26	27	28
29	30					

JULY 2025

S	M	T	W	T	F	S
		1	2	3	4	5
6	7	8	9	10	11	12
13	14	15	16	17	18	19
20	21	22	23	24	25	26
27	28	29	30	31		

AUGUST 2025

S	M	T	W	T	F	S
					1	2
3	4	5	6	7	8	9
10	11	12	13	14	15	16
17	18	19	20	21	22	23
$24/31$	25	26	27	28	29	30

SEPTEMBER 2025

S	M	T	W	T	F	S
	1	2	3	4	5	6
7	8	9	10	11	12	13
14	15	16	17	18	19	20
21	22	23	24	25	26	27
28	29	30				

OCTOBER 2025

S	M	T	W	T	F	S
			1	2	3	4
5	6	7	8	9	10	11
12	13	14	15	16	17	18
19	20	21	22	23	24	25
26	27	28	29	30	31	

NOVEMBER 2025

S	M	T	W	T	F	S
						1
2	3	4	5	6	7	8
9	10	11	12	13	14	15
16	17	18	19	20	21	22
$23/30$	24	25	26	27	28	29

DECEMBER 2025

S	M	T	W	T	F	S
	1	2	3	4	5	6
7	8	9	10	11	12	13
14	15	16	17	18	19	20
21	22	23	24	25	26	27
28	29	30	31			

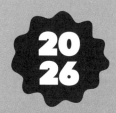 AT A GLANCE

JANUARY 2026

S	M	T	W	T	F	S
				1	2	3
4	5	6	7	8	9	10
11	12	13	14	15	16	17
18	19	20	21	22	23	24
25	26	27	28	29	30	31

FEBRUARY 2026

S	M	T	W	T	F	S
1	2	3	4	5	6	7
8	9	10	11	12	13	14
15	16	17	18	19	20	21
22	23	24	25	26	27	28

MARCH 2026

S	M	T	W	T	F	S
1	2	3	4	5	6	7
8	9	10	11	12	13	14
15	16	17	18	19	20	21
22	23	24	25	26	27	28
29	30	31				

APRIL 2026

S	M	T	W	T	F	S
			1	2	3	4
5	6	7	8	9	10	11
12	13	14	15	16	17	18
19	20	21	22	23	24	25
26	27	28	29	30		

MAY 2026

S	M	T	W	T	F	S
					1	2
3	4	5	6	7	8	9
10	11	12	13	14	15	16
17	18	19	20	21	22	23
$^{24}/_{31}$	25	26	27	28	29	30

JUNE 2026

S	M	T	W	T	F	S
	1	2	3	4	5	6
7	8	9	10	11	12	13
14	15	16	17	18	19	20
21	22	23	24	25	26	27
28	29	30				

JULY 2026

S	M	T	W	T	F	S
			1	2	3	4
5	6	7	8	9	10	11
12	13	14	15	16	17	18
19	20	21	22	23	24	25
26	27	28	29	30	31	

AUGUST 2026

S	M	T	W	T	F	S
						1
2	3	4	5	6	7	8
9	10	11	12	13	14	15
16	17	18	19	20	21	22
$^{23}/_{30}$	$^{24}/_{31}$	25	26	27	28	29

SEPTEMBER 2026

S	M	T	W	T	F	S
		1	2	3	4	5
6	7	8	9	10	11	12
13	14	15	16	17	18	19
20	21	22	23	24	25	26
27	28	29	30			

OCTOBER 2026

S	M	T	W	T	F	S
				1	2	3
4	5	6	7	8	9	10
11	12	13	14	15	16	17
18	19	20	21	22	23	24
25	26	27	28	29	30	31

NOVEMBER 2026

S	M	T	W	T	F	S
1	2	3	4	5	6	7
8	9	10	11	12	13	14
15	16	17	18	19	20	21
22	23	24	25	26	27	28
29	30					

DECEMBER 2026

S	M	T	W	T	F	S
		1	2	3	4	5
6	7	8	9	10	11	12
13	14	15	16	17	18	19
20	21	22	23	24	25	26
27	28	29	30	31		

MONTHLY GOALS & SHIT

FUCKING FITNESS GOALS

ANOTHER DAMN LIST

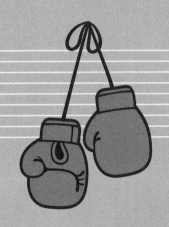

GET IT
FUCKING
GOING

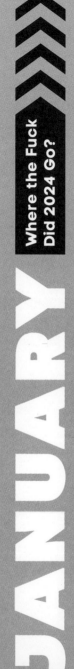

Where the Fuck Did 2024 Go?

JANUARY

20 25

SUNDAY	MONDAY	TUESDAY
29	30	31
5	6	7
12	13	14
19	20	21
	Martin Luther King Jr. Day	
26	27	28
Australia Day (AUS)		

WEDNESDAY	THURSDAY	FRIDAY	SATURDAY
1 New Year's Day	2 Day after New Year's Day (NZ, SCT)	3	4
8	9	10	11
15	16	17	18
22	23	24	25
29 Lunar New Year	30	31	1

SWEAT OUT THE BULLSHIT

DAY	ACTIVITY	TIME	DISTANCE	WEIGHT LIFTED	SETS/ REPS	

IT'S ONLY A HABIT IF YOU FUCKING DO IT.

HABIT	M	T	W	TH	F	SA	SU
Drink enough water, bitch.							

DECEMBER/JANUARY

MONDAY
30

TUESDAY
31
New Year's Eve

WEDNESDAY
1
New Year's Day

RESOLUTION #1: DON'T BE AN ASSHOLE.

THURSDAY
2
Day after New Year's Day (NZ, SCT)

THE LAST OF THE DAMN HOLIDAYS. SHIT.

FRIDAY
3

SATURDAY
4

SUNDAY
5

NOTEWORTHY SHIT

SWEAT OUT THE BULLSHIT

DAY	ACTIVITY	TIME	DISTANCE	WEIGHT LIFTED	SETS/ REPS	

IT'S ONLY A HABIT IF YOU FUCKING DO IT.

HABIT	M	T	W	TH	F	SA	SU
Drink enough water, bitch.							

JANUARY

MONDAY »
6

TUESDAY »
7

WEDNESDAY »
8

THURSDAY »
9

FRIDAY »
10

SATURDAY »
11

SUNDAY »
12

NOTEWORTHY SHIT

SWEAT OUT THE BULLSHIT

DAY	ACTIVITY	TIME	DISTANCE	WEIGHT LIFTED	SETS/ REPS	

IT'S ONLY A HABIT IF YOU FUCKING DO IT.

HABIT	M	T	W	TH	F	SA	SU
Drink enough water, bitch.							

JANUARY

MONDAY »
13

TUESDAY »
14

IT'S STILL FUCKING FREEZING OUTSIDE!

WEDNESDAY »
15

THURSDAY »
16

FRIDAY »
17

SATURDAY »
18

SUNDAY »
19

NOTEWORTHY SHIT

SWEAT OUT THE BULLSHIT

DAY	ACTIVITY	TIME	DISTANCE	WEIGHT LIFTED	SETS/ REPS	

IT'S ONLY A HABIT IF YOU FUCKING DO IT.

HABIT	M	T	W	TH	F	SA	SU
Drink enough water, bitch.							

JANUARY

MONDAY
Martin Luther King Jr. Day
20

TUESDAY
21

ALREADY FUCKED UP THOSE RESOLUTIONS.

WEDNESDAY
22

THURSDAY
23

FRIDAY
24

SATURDAY
25

SUNDAY
Australia Day (AUS)
26

NOTEWORTHY SHIT

SWEAT OUT THE BULLSHIT

DAY	ACTIVITY	TIME	DISTANCE	WEIGHT LIFTED	SETS/ REPS	

IT'S ONLY A HABIT IF YOU FUCKING DO IT.

HABIT	M	T	W	TH	F	SA	SU
Drink enough water, bitch.							

JANUARY/FEBRUARY

MONDAY »
27

TUESDAY »
28

WEDNESDAY » Lunar New Year
29

THURSDAY »
30

FRIDAY »
31

SATURDAY »
1

SUNDAY » Groundhog Day
2

RODENTS DON'T KNOW SHIT ABOUT WEATHER.

NOTEWORTHY SHIT

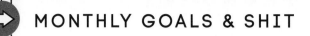 MONTHLY GOALS & SHIT

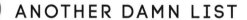 FUCKING FITNESS GOALS

ANOTHER DAMN LIST

DON'T SWEAT THE SMALL SHIT

FEBRUARY

At Least There's Fucking Chocolate.

2025

SUNDAY	MONDAY	TUESDAY
26	27	28
2 Groundhog Day	3	4
9	10	11
16	17 Presidents' Day	18
23	24	25

WEDNESDAY	THURSDAY	FRIDAY	SATURDAY
29	30	31	1
5	6 Waitangi Day (NZ)	7	8
12 Abraham Lincoln's Birthday	13	14 Valentine's Day	15
19	20	21	22
26	27	28 Ramadan begins	1

SWEAT OUT THE BULLSHIT

DAY	ACTIVITY	TIME	DISTANCE	WEIGHT LIFTED	SETS/ REPS	

IT'S ONLY A HABIT IF YOU FUCKING DO IT.

HABIT	M	T	W	TH	F	SA	SU
Drink enough water, bitch.							

FEBRUARY

MONDAY »
3

TUESDAY »
4

IT'S A LITTLE EARLY FOR ALL THIS RED AND PINK SHIT.

WEDNESDAY »
5

Waitangi Day (NZ)

THURSDAY »
6

FRIDAY »
7

SATURDAY »
8

SUNDAY »
9

NOTEWORTHY SHIT

SWEAT OUT THE BULLSHIT

DAY	ACTIVITY	TIME	DISTANCE	WEIGHT LIFTED	SETS/ REPS	

IT'S ONLY A HABIT IF YOU FUCKING DO IT.

HABIT	M	T	W	TH	F	SA	SU
Drink enough water, bitch.							

FEBRUARY

MONDAY »
10

TUESDAY »
11

WEDNESDAY »   Abraham Lincoln's Birthday
12

THURSDAY »
13

FRIDAY »   Valentine's Day
14

CUPID IS A LYING BASTARD.

SATURDAY »   **SUNDAY** »
15   16

NOTEWORTHY SHIT

SWEAT OUT THE BULLSHIT

DAY	ACTIVITY	TIME	DISTANCE	WEIGHT LIFTED	SETS/ REPS	

IT'S ONLY A HABIT IF YOU FUCKING DO IT.

HABIT	M	T	W	TH	F	SA	SU
Drink enough water, bitch.							

FEBRUARY

MONDAY »
17

TUESDAY »
18

WEDNESDAY »
19

THURSDAY »
20

FRIDAY »
21

SATURDAY »
22

SUNDAY »
23

NOTEWORTHY SHIT

SWEAT OUT THE BULLSHIT

DAY	ACTIVITY	TIME	DISTANCE	WEIGHT LIFTED	SETS/ REPS	

IT'S ONLY A HABIT IF YOU FUCKING DO IT.

HABIT	M	T	W	TH	F	SA	SU
Drink enough water, bitch.							

FEBRUARY/MARCH

MONDAY »
24

OWN THIS WEEK LIKE A BOSS-ASS BITCH!

TUESDAY »
25

WEDNESDAY »
26

THURSDAY »
27

FRIDAY »
28

Ramadan begins

SATURDAY »
1

SUNDAY »
2

NOTEWORTHY SHIT

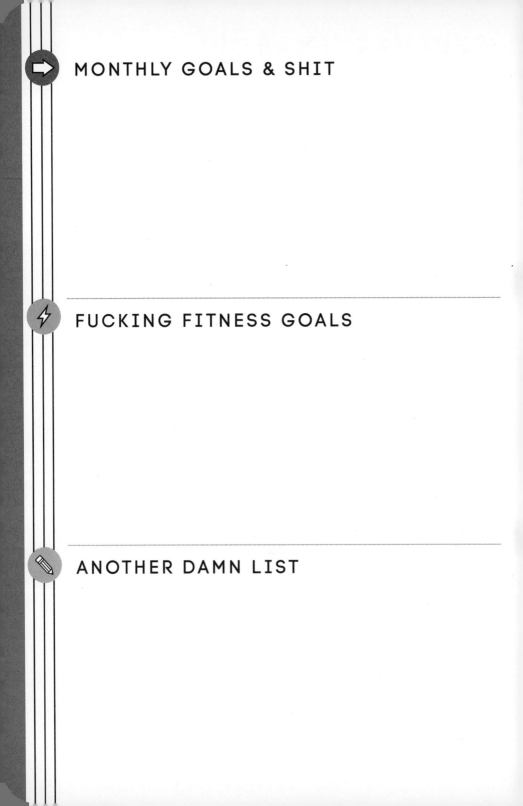

➡ MONTHLY GOALS & SHIT

⚡ FUCKING FITNESS GOALS

✎ ANOTHER DAMN LIST

TOO FUCKING FIT TO QUIT

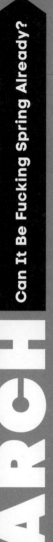

MARCH

Can It Be Fucking Spring Already?

2025

SUNDAY	MONDAY	TUESDAY
23	24	25
2	3	4
9 Daylight Saving Time begins (USA, CAN)	10 Public Holiday (AUS: ACT, SA, TAS, VIC)	11
16	17 St. Patrick's Day	18
23	24	25
30 Eid al-Fitr begins; Mothering Sunday (UK)	31	

WEDNESDAY	THURSDAY	FRIDAY	SATURDAY
26	27	28	1
5 Ash Wednesday (Lent begins)	6	7	8 International Women's Day
12	13 Purim begins	14	15
19	20 Spring begins (Northern Hemisphere)	21	22
26	27	28	29

SWEAT OUT THE BULLSHIT

DAY	ACTIVITY	TIME	DISTANCE	WEIGHT LIFTED	SETS/ REPS	

IT'S ONLY A HABIT IF YOU FUCKING DO IT.

HABIT	M	T	W	TH	F	SA	SU
Drink enough water, bitch.							

MARCH

MONDAY »
3

TUESDAY »
4

WEDNESDAY »
5
Ash Wednesday (Lent begins)

THURSDAY »
6

FRIDAY »
7

SATURDAY »
8
International Women's Day

FUCK THE PATRIARCHY.

SUNDAY »
9
Daylight Saving Time begins (USA, CAN)

GREAT, ONE LESS FUCKING HOUR OF SLEEP.

NOTEWORTHY SHIT

SWEAT OUT THE BULLSHIT

DAY	ACTIVITY	TIME	DISTANCE	WEIGHT LIFTED	SETS/ REPS	

IT'S ONLY A HABIT IF YOU FUCKING DO IT.

HABIT	M	T	W	TH	F	SA	SU
Drink enough water, bitch.							

MARCH

MONDAY »
10

Public Holiday
(AUS: ACT, SA, TAS, VIC)

TUESDAY »
11

WEDNESDAY »
12

THURSDAY »
13

Purim begins

FRIDAY »
14

SATURDAY »
15

SUNDAY »
16

NOTEWORTHY SHIT

SWEAT OUT THE BULLSHIT

DAY	ACTIVITY	TIME	DISTANCE	WEIGHT LIFTED	SETS/ REPS	

IT'S ONLY A HABIT IF YOU FUCKING DO IT.

HABIT	M	T	W	TH	F	SA	SU
Drink enough water, bitch.							

MARCH

MONDAY »
17

LEPRECHAUNS ARE NOT FUCKING REAL.

TUESDAY »
18

WEDNESDAY »
19

Spring begins (Northern Hemisphere)

THURSDAY »
20

FLOWERS AREN'T WORTH THIS ALLERGY SHIT.

FRIDAY »
21

SATURDAY »
22

SUNDAY »
23

NOTEWORTHY SHIT

SWEAT OUT THE BULLSHIT

DAY	ACTIVITY	TIME	DISTANCE	WEIGHT LIFTED	SETS/ REPS	

IT'S ONLY A HABIT IF YOU FUCKING DO IT.

HABIT	M	T	W	TH	F	SA	SU
Drink enough water, bitch.							

MARCH

24

25

26

27

28

29

30

Eid al-Fitr begins;
Mothering Sunday (UK)

NOTEWORTHY SHIT

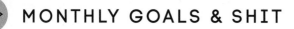

MONTHLY GOALS & SHIT

FUCKING FITNESS GOALS

ANOTHER DAMN LIST

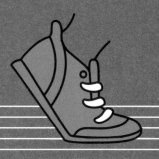

LIKE A
FUCKING
BOSS

SUNDAY	MONDAY	TUESDAY
30	31	1 April Fools' Day
6	7	8
13 Palm Sunday	14	15 Tax Day
20 Easter	21 Easter Monday (AUS, CAN, NZ, UK except SCT)	22 Earth Day
27	28 Workers' Memorial Day (UK)	29

WEDNESDAY	THURSDAY	FRIDAY	SATURDAY
2	3	4	5
9	10	11	12 Passover begins
16	17	18 Good Friday	19
23	24	25 Anzac Day (AUS, NZ)	26
30	1	2	3

SWEAT OUT THE BULLSHIT

DAY	ACTIVITY	TIME	DISTANCE	WEIGHT LIFTED	SETS/ REPS	

IT'S ONLY A HABIT IF YOU FUCKING DO IT.

HABIT	M	T	W	TH	F	SA	SU
Drink enough water, bitch.							

MARCH/APRIL

MONDAY »
31

TUESDAY »
1

April Fools' Day

WATCH YOUR DAMN BACK.

WEDNESDAY »
2

THURSDAY »
3

FRIDAY »
4

SATURDAY »
5

SUNDAY »
6

NOTEWORTHY SHIT

SWEAT OUT THE BULLSHIT

DAY	ACTIVITY	TIME	DISTANCE	WEIGHT LIFTED	SETS/ REPS	

IT'S ONLY A HABIT IF YOU FUCKING DO IT.

HABIT	M	T	W	TH	F	SA	SU
Drink enough water, bitch.							

APRIL

MONDAY »
7

TUESDAY »
8

WEDNESDAY »
9

THURSDAY »
10

CLEAN YOUR DAMN HOUSE.

FRIDAY »
11

SATURDAY »   Passover begins
12

SUNDAY »   Palm Sunday
13

NOTEWORTHY SHIT

SWEAT OUT THE BULLSHIT

DAY	ACTIVITY	TIME	DISTANCE	WEIGHT LIFTED	SETS/ REPS	

IT'S ONLY A HABIT IF YOU FUCKING DO IT.

HABIT	M	T	W	TH	F	SA	SU
Drink enough water, bitch.							

APRIL

Tax Day

PONY UP, BITCH! IT'S TAX DAY.

Good Friday

Easter

NOTEWORTHY SHIT

SWEAT OUT THE BULLSHIT

DAY	ACTIVITY	TIME	DISTANCE	WEIGHT LIFTED	SETS/ REPS	

IT'S ONLY A HABIT IF YOU FUCKING DO IT.

HABIT	M	T	W	TH	F	SA	SU
Drink enough water, bitch.							

APRIL

Easter Monday
(AUS, CAN, NZ, UK except SCT)

TUESDAY ≫

22

Earth Day

REDUCE, REUSE, RECYCLE, ASSHOLES!

WEDNESDAY ≫

23

THURSDAY ≫

24

FRIDAY ≫

25

Anzac Day (AUS, NZ)

SATURDAY ≫

26

SUNDAY ≫

27

NOTEWORTHY SHIT

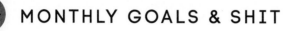

MONTHLY GOALS & SHIT

FUCKING FITNESS GOALS

ANOTHER DAMN LIST

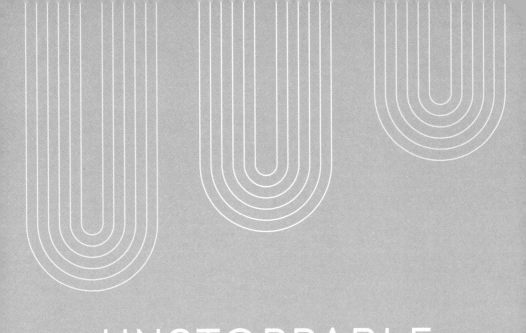

UNSTOPPABLE
AS HELL

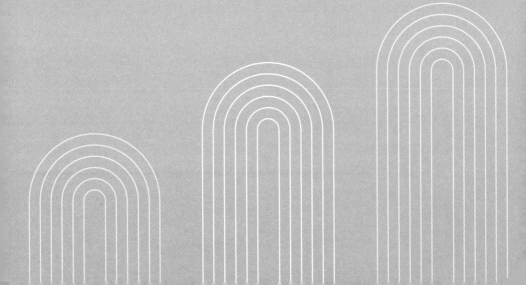

MAY

Fucking Graduation Season (woo)!

2025

SUNDAY	MONDAY	TUESDAY
27	28	29
4	5 Cinco de Mayo	6
11 Mother's Day (USA, AUS, CAN, NZ)	12	13
18	19 Victoria Day (CAN)	20
25	26 Memorial Day (USA); Spring Bank Holiday (UK)	27

WEDNESDAY	THURSDAY	FRIDAY	SATURDAY
30	1	2	3
7	8	9	10
14	15	16	17 Armed Forces Day
21	22	23	24
28	29	30	31

SWEAT OUT THE BULLSHIT

DAY	ACTIVITY	TIME	DISTANCE	WEIGHT LIFTED	SETS/ REPS	

IT'S ONLY A HABIT IF YOU FUCKING DO IT.

HABIT	M	T	W	TH	F	SA	SU
Drink enough water, bitch.							

APRIL/MAY

MONDAY »
28

TUESDAY »
29

WEDNESDAY »
30

THURSDAY »
1

FRIDAY »
2

SATURDAY »
3

SUNDAY »
4

MAY THE FUCKING FOURTH BE WITH YOU.

NOTEWORTHY SHIT

SWEAT OUT THE BULLSHIT

DAY	ACTIVITY	TIME	DISTANCE	WEIGHT LIFTED	SETS/ REPS	

IT'S ONLY A HABIT IF YOU FUCKING DO IT.

HABIT	M	T	W	TH	F	SA	SU
Drink enough water, bitch.							

MAY

MONDAY 〉〉   Cinco de Mayo

5

TUESDAY 〉〉

6

WEDNESDAY 〉〉

7

THURSDAY 〉〉

8

FRIDAY 〉〉

9

SATURDAY 〉〉

10

SUNDAY 〉〉   Mother's Day
(USA, AUS, CAN, NZ)

11

TREAT YOUR MOM LIKE A FUCKING QUEEN.

NOTEWORTHY SHIT

SWEAT OUT THE BULLSHIT

DAY	ACTIVITY	TIME	DISTANCE	WEIGHT LIFTED	SETS/ REPS	

IT'S ONLY A HABIT IF YOU FUCKING DO IT.

HABIT	M	T	W	TH	F	SA	SU
Drink enough water, bitch.							

MAY

MONDAY
12

TUESDAY
13

WEDNESDAY
14

THURSDAY
15

FRIDAY
16

SATURDAY   Armed Forces Day   **SUNDAY**
17   18

NOTEWORTHY SHIT

SWEAT OUT THE BULLSHIT

DAY	ACTIVITY	TIME	DISTANCE	WEIGHT LIFTED	SETS/ REPS	

IT'S ONLY A HABIT IF YOU FUCKING DO IT.

HABIT	M	T	W	TH	F	SA	SU
Drink enough water, bitch.							

MAY

MONDAY 19
Victoria Day (CAN)

TUESDAY 20

WEDNESDAY 21

THURSDAY 22

FRIDAY 23

HELL YEAH, THREE-DAY WEEKEND!

SATURDAY 24

SUNDAY 25

NOTEWORTHY SHIT

SWEAT OUT THE BULLSHIT

DAY	ACTIVITY	TIME	DISTANCE	WEIGHT LIFTED	SETS/ REPS	

IT'S ONLY A HABIT IF YOU FUCKING DO IT.

HABIT	M	T	W	TH	F	SA	SU
Drink enough water, bitch.							

MAY/JUNE

MONDAY 〉〉

26

Memorial Day (USA);
Spring Bank Holiday (UK)

TUESDAY 〉〉

27

WEDNESDAY 〉〉

28

THURSDAY 〉〉

29

FRIDAY 〉〉

30

SATURDAY 〉〉

31

SUNDAY 〉〉

1

Shavuot begins

NOTEWORTHY SHIT

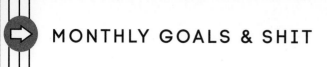

MONTHLY GOALS & SHIT

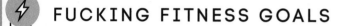

FUCKING FITNESS GOALS

ANOTHER DAMN LIST

BELIEVE IT

AND

F*CKING

ACHIEVE IT

SUNDAY	MONDAY	TUESDAY
1 Shavuot begins	2	3
8	9	10
15 Father's Day (USA, CAN, UK)	16	17
22	23	24
29	30	1

WEDNESDAY	THURSDAY	FRIDAY	SATURDAY
4	5	6 Eid al-Adha begins	7
11	12	13	14 Flag Day
18	19 Juneteenth	20 Summer begins (Northern Hemisphere)	21
25	26	27	28
2	3	4	5

SWEAT OUT THE BULLSHIT

DAY	ACTIVITY	TIME	DISTANCE	WEIGHT LIFTED	SETS/ REPS	

IT'S ONLY A HABIT IF YOU FUCKING DO IT.

HABIT	M	T	W	TH	F	SA	SU
Drink enough water, bitch.							

JUNE

MONDAY »
2

TUESDAY »
3

WEDNESDAY »
4

THURSDAY »
5

ALMOST FRI-FUCKING-YAY!

Eid al-Adha begins

FRIDAY »
6

SATURDAY »
7

SUNDAY »
8

NOTEWORTHY SHIT

SWEAT OUT THE BULLSHIT

DAY	ACTIVITY	TIME	DISTANCE	WEIGHT LIFTED	SETS/ REPS	

IT'S ONLY A HABIT IF YOU FUCKING DO IT.

HABIT	M	T	W	TH	F	SA	SU
Drink enough water, bitch.							

JUNE

MONDAY »

9

TUESDAY »

10

WEDNESDAY »

11

THURSDAY »

12

FRIDAY »

13

GOOD FUCKING LUCK!

SATURDAY »   Flag Day

14

SUNDAY »   Father's Day
(USA, CAN, UK)

15

NOTE: DADS ARE THE SHIT.

NOTEWORTHY SHIT

SWEAT OUT THE BULLSHIT

DAY	ACTIVITY	TIME	DISTANCE	WEIGHT LIFTED	SETS/ REPS	

IT'S ONLY A HABIT IF YOU FUCKING DO IT.

HABIT	M	T	W	TH	F	SA	SU
Drink enough water, bitch.							

JUNE

MONDAY »
16

TUESDAY »
17

WEDNESDAY »
18

THURSDAY »   Juneteenth
19

FRIDAY »   Summer begins
20   (Northern Hemisphere)

LONGEST. DAY. OF. THE. DAMN. YEAR.

SATURDAY » | **SUNDAY** »
21 | 22

NOTEWORTHY SHIT

SWEAT OUT THE BULLSHIT

DAY	ACTIVITY	TIME	DISTANCE	WEIGHT LIFTED	SETS/ REPS	

IT'S ONLY A HABIT IF YOU FUCKING DO IT.

HABIT	M	T	W	TH	F	SA	SU
Drink enough water, bitch.							

JUNE

MONDAY
23

TUESDAY
24

WEDNESDAY
25

THURSDAY
26

FRIDAY
27

SATURDAY
28

SUNDAY
29

NOTEWORTHY SHIT

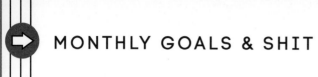 MONTHLY GOALS & SHIT

 FUCKING FITNESS GOALS

ANOTHER DAMN LIST

GET
SHIT
DONE

JULY 2025

Get Some Fucking Sunshine!

SUNDAY	MONDAY	TUESDAY
29	30	1 Canada Day (CAN)
6	7	8
13	14	15
20	21	22
27	28	29

WEDNESDAY	THURSDAY	FRIDAY	SATURDAY
2	3	4 Independence Day	5
9	10	11	12 Orangemen's Day— Battle of the Boyne (NIR)
16	17	18	19
23	24	25	26
30	31	1	2

SWEAT OUT THE BULLSHIT

DAY	ACTIVITY	TIME	DISTANCE	WEIGHT LIFTED	SETS/ REPS	

IT'S ONLY A HABIT IF YOU FUCKING DO IT.

HABIT	M	T	W	TH	F	SA	SU
Drink enough water, bitch.							

JUNE/JULY

MONDAY »
30

TUESDAY »   Canada Day (CAN)
1

WEDNESDAY »
2

THURSDAY »
3

FRIDAY »   Independence Day
4

SNAP, CRACKLE, POP THAT SHIT!

SATURDAY »   **SUNDAY** »
5   6

NOTEWORTHY SHIT

SWEAT OUT THE BULLSHIT

DAY	ACTIVITY	TIME	DISTANCE	WEIGHT LIFTED	SETS/ REPS	

IT'S ONLY A HABIT IF YOU FUCKING DO IT.

HABIT	M	T	W	TH	F	SA	SU
Drink enough water, bitch.							

JULY

MONDAY »
7

TUESDAY »
8

WEDNESDAY »
9

THURSDAY »
10

FRIDAY »
11

SATURDAY »   Orangemen's Day—   **SUNDAY** »
12   Battle of the Boyne (NIR)   13

NOTEWORTHY SHIT

FITNESS LOG

SWEAT OUT THE BULLSHIT

DAY	ACTIVITY	TIME	DISTANCE	WEIGHT LIFTED	SETS/ REPS	

IT'S ONLY A HABIT IF YOU FUCKING DO IT.

HABIT	M	T	W	TH	F	SA	SU
Drink enough water, bitch.							

JULY

MONDAY »
14

TUESDAY »
15

WEDNESDAY »
16

THURSDAY »
17

FRIDAY »
18

COOL IT WITH THE DAMN FIREWORKS, PEOPLE!

SATURDAY »
19

SUNDAY »
20

NOTEWORTHY SHIT

SWEAT OUT THE BULLSHIT

DAY	ACTIVITY	TIME	DISTANCE	WEIGHT LIFTED	SETS/ REPS	

IT'S ONLY A HABIT IF YOU FUCKING DO IT.

HABIT	M	T	W	TH	F	SA	SU
Drink enough water, bitch.							

JULY

TUESDAY »
22

WEDNESDAY »
23

THURSDAY »
24

FRIDAY »
25

SATURDAY »
26

SUNDAY »
27

NOTEWORTHY SHIT

FITNESS LOG

SWEAT OUT THE BULLSHIT

DAY	ACTIVITY	TIME	DISTANCE	WEIGHT LIFTED	SETS/ REPS	

IT'S ONLY A HABIT IF YOU FUCKING DO IT.

HABIT	M	T	W	TH	F	SA	SU
Drink enough water, bitch.							

JULY/AUGUST

MONDAY >>
28

BRING ON THOSE SEXY-AS-HELL WATCH TANS!

TUESDAY >>
29

WEDNESDAY >>
30

THURSDAY >>
31

FRIDAY >>
1

SATURDAY >>
2

SUNDAY >>
3

NOTEWORTHY SHIT

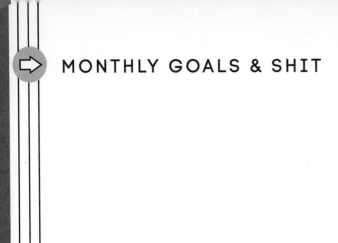

MONTHLY GOALS & SHIT

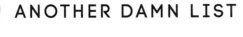

FUCKING FITNESS GOALS

✏ ANOTHER DAMN LIST

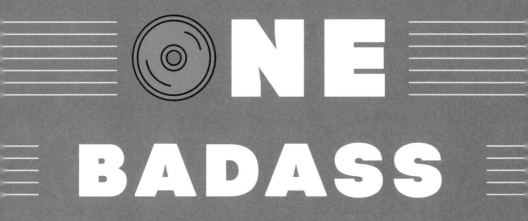

ONE
BADASS
MOTHERFUCKER

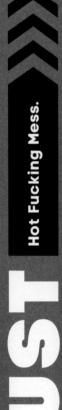

AUGUST

Hot Fucking Mess.

20 25

SUNDAY	MONDAY	TUESDAY
27	28	29
3	4 Summer Bank Holiday (SCT)	5
10	11	12
17	18	19
24	25 Summer Bank Holiday (UK except SCT)	26
31		

WEDNESDAY	THURSDAY	FRIDAY	SATURDAY
30	31	1	2
6	7	8	9
13	14	15	16
20	21	22	23
27	28	29	30

SWEAT OUT THE BULLSHIT

DAY	ACTIVITY	TIME	DISTANCE	WEIGHT LIFTED	SETS/ REPS	

IT'S ONLY A HABIT IF YOU FUCKING DO IT.

HABIT	M	T	W	TH	F	SA	SU
Drink enough water, bitch.							

AUGUST

MONDAY »
4

NAMA-STAY THE FUCK IN BED.

TUESDAY »
5

WEDNESDAY »
6

THURSDAY »
7

FRIDAY »
8

SATURDAY »
9

SUNDAY »
10

NOTEWORTHY SHIT

SWEAT OUT THE BULLSHIT

DAY	ACTIVITY	TIME	DISTANCE	WEIGHT LIFTED	SETS/ REPS	

IT'S ONLY A HABIT IF YOU FUCKING DO IT.

HABIT	M	T	W	TH	F	SA	SU
Drink enough water, bitch.							

AUGUST

MONDAY »
11

TUESDAY »
12

WEDNESDAY »
13

THURSDAY »
14

GET YOUR ASS TO THE DAMN POOL.

FRIDAY »
15

SATURDAY »
16

SUNDAY »
17

NOTEWORTHY SHIT

SWEAT OUT THE BULLSHIT

DAY	ACTIVITY	TIME	DISTANCE	WEIGHT LIFTED	SETS/ REPS	

IT'S ONLY A HABIT IF YOU FUCKING DO IT.

HABIT	M	T	W	TH	F	SA	SU
Drink enough water, bitch.							

AUGUST

MONDAY »
18

TUESDAY »
19

WEDNESDAY »
20

HELL YEAH, HUMP DAAAYYY!

THURSDAY »
21

FRIDAY »
22

SATURDAY »
23

SUNDAY »
24

NOTEWORTHY SHIT

SWEAT OUT THE BULLSHIT

DAY	ACTIVITY	TIME	DISTANCE	WEIGHT LIFTED	SETS/ REPS	

IT'S ONLY A HABIT IF YOU FUCKING DO IT.

HABIT	M	T	W	TH	F	SA	SU
Drink enough water, bitch.							

AUGUST

MONDAY ❯❯
25

Summer Bank Holiday
(UK except SCT)

TUESDAY ❯❯
26

WEDNESDAY ❯❯
27

THURSDAY ❯❯
28

FRIDAY ❯❯
29

PEACE OUT, BITCHES! THREE-DAY WEEKEND!

SATURDAY ❯❯
30

SUNDAY ❯❯
31

NOTEWORTHY SHIT

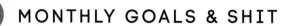

MONTHLY GOALS & SHIT

FUCKING FITNESS GOALS

ANOTHER DAMN LIST

MIND OVER FUCKING MATTER

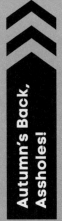

Autumn's Back, Assholes!

SEPTEMBER

2025

SUNDAY	MONDAY	TUESDAY
31	1 Labor Day (USA, CAN)	2
7 Father's Day (AUS, NZ)	8	9
14	15	16
21	22 Rosh Hashanah begins; Autumn begins (Northern Hemisphere)	23
28	29	30

WEDNESDAY	THURSDAY	FRIDAY	SATURDAY
3	4	5	6
10	11 Patriot Day	12	13
17	18	19	20
24	25	26	27
1	2	3	4

SWEAT OUT THE BULLSHIT

DAY	ACTIVITY	TIME	DISTANCE	WEIGHT LIFTED	SETS/ REPS	

IT'S ONLY A HABIT IF YOU FUCKING DO IT.

HABIT	M	T	W	TH	F	SA	SU
Drink enough water, bitch.							

SEPTEMBER

MONDAY 〉〉 Labor Day (USA, CAN)

1

TUESDAY 〉〉

2

WEDNESDAY 〉〉

3

THURSDAY 〉〉

4

FRIDAY 〉〉

5

SATURDAY 〉〉

6

SUNDAY 〉〉 Father's Day (AUS, NZ)

7

NOTEWORTHY SHIT

SWEAT OUT THE BULLSHIT

DAY	ACTIVITY	TIME	DISTANCE	WEIGHT LIFTED	SETS/ REPS	

IT'S ONLY A HABIT IF YOU FUCKING DO IT.

HABIT	M	T	W	TH	F	SA	SU
Drink enough water, bitch.							

SEPTEMBER

MONDAY
8

TUESDAY
9

WEDNESDAY
10

THURSDAY
11   Patriot Day

FRIDAY
12

SATURDAY | **SUNDAY**
13 | 14

GO CARVE SOME DAMN PUMPKINS.

NOTEWORTHY SHIT

SWEAT OUT THE BULLSHIT

DAY	ACTIVITY	TIME	DISTANCE	WEIGHT LIFTED	SETS/ REPS	

IT'S ONLY A HABIT IF YOU FUCKING DO IT.

HABIT	M	T	W	TH	F	SA	SU
Drink enough water, bitch.							

SEPTEMBER

MONDAY 〉
15

TUESDAY 〉
16

WEDNESDAY 〉
17

THURSDAY 〉
18

FRIDAY 〉
19

SATURDAY 〉
20

SUNDAY 〉
21

NOTEWORTHY SHIT

SWEAT OUT THE BULLSHIT

DAY	ACTIVITY	TIME	DISTANCE	WEIGHT LIFTED	SETS/ REPS	

IT'S ONLY A HABIT IF YOU FUCKING DO IT.

HABIT	M	T	W	TH	F	SA	SU
Drink enough water, bitch.							

SEPTEMBER

MONDAY

22

Rosh Hashanah begins;
Autumn begins
(Northern Hemisphere)

TUESDAY

23

WEDNESDAY

24

THURSDAY

25

FRIDAY

26

OH, COOL. FUCKING LEAVES EVERYWHERE.

SATURDAY

27

SUNDAY

28

NOTEWORTHY SHIT

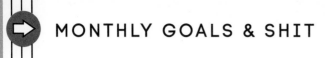 MONTHLY GOALS & SHIT

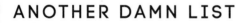 FUCKING FITNESS GOALS

ANOTHER DAMN LIST

PRACTICE MAKES DAMN PROGRESS

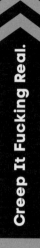

OCTOBER

Creep It Fucking Real.

SUNDAY	MONDAY	TUESDAY
28	29	30
5	6	7
	Sukkot begins	
12	13	14
	Columbus Day (USA); Indigenous Peoples' Day (USA); Thanksgiving Day (CAN)	
19	20	21
	Diwali begins	
26	27	28

20
25

WEDNESDAY	THURSDAY	FRIDAY	SATURDAY
1 Yom Kippur begins	2	3	4
8	9	10	11
15	16	17	18
22	23	24	25
29	30	31 Halloween	1

SWEAT OUT THE BULLSHIT

DAY	ACTIVITY	TIME	DISTANCE	WEIGHT LIFTED	SETS/ REPS	

IT'S ONLY A HABIT IF YOU FUCKING DO IT.

HABIT	M	T	W	TH	F	SA	SU
Drink enough water, bitch.							

SEPTEMBER/OCTOBER

MONDAY
29

TUESDAY
30

WEDNESDAY   Yom Kippur begins
1

THURSDAY
2

IT'S NEVER TOO EARLY TO SCARE THE SHIT OUT OF SOMEONE.

FRIDAY
3

SATURDAY   **SUNDAY**
4   5

NOTEWORTHY SHIT

SWEAT OUT THE BULLSHIT

DAY	ACTIVITY	TIME	DISTANCE	WEIGHT LIFTED	SETS/ REPS	

IT'S ONLY A HABIT IF YOU FUCKING DO IT.

HABIT	M	T	W	TH	F	SA	SU
Drink enough water, bitch.							

OCTOBER

MONDAY 〉

6

Sukkot begins

TUESDAY 〉

7

WEDNESDAY 〉

8

THURSDAY 〉

9

FRIDAY 〉

10

SATURDAY 〉

11

SUNDAY 〉

12

NOTEWORTHY SHIT

SWEAT OUT THE BULLSHIT

DAY	ACTIVITY	TIME	DISTANCE	WEIGHT LIFTED	SETS/ REPS	

IT'S ONLY A HABIT IF YOU FUCKING DO IT.

HABIT	M	T	W	TH	F	SA	SU
Drink enough water, bitch.							

OCTOBER

13

Columbus Day (USA);
Indigenous Peoples' Day (USA);
Thanksgiving Day (CAN)

HEY CANADA, HAPPY FUCKING THANKSGIVING.

TUESDAY >>
14

WEDNESDAY >>
15

THURSDAY >>
16

FRIDAY >>
17

SATURDAY >>
18

SUNDAY >>
19

NOTEWORTHY SHIT

SWEAT OUT THE BULLSHIT

DAY	ACTIVITY	TIME	DISTANCE	WEIGHT LIFTED	SETS/ REPS	

IT'S ONLY A HABIT IF YOU FUCKING DO IT.

HABIT	M	T	W	TH	F	SA	SU
Drink enough water, bitch.							

OCTOBER

Diwali begins

MONDAY »
20

TUESDAY »
21

WEDNESDAY »
22

THURSDAY »
23

FRIDAY »
24

SATURDAY »
25

SUNDAY »
26

CUE THE SHITTY
HALLOWEEN COSTUME SCRAMBLE.

NOTEWORTHY SHIT

SWEAT OUT THE BULLSHIT

DAY	ACTIVITY	TIME	DISTANCE	WEIGHT LIFTED	SETS/ REPS	

IT'S ONLY A HABIT IF YOU FUCKING DO IT.

HABIT	M	T	W	TH	F	SA	SU
Drink enough water, bitch.							

OCTOBER/NOVEMBER

MONDAY
27

TUESDAY
28

WEDNESDAY
29

THURSDAY
30

FRIDAY   Halloween
31

TREAT YOUR BADASS SELF!

SATURDAY   **SUNDAY**   Daylight Saving
1   2   Time ends (USA, CAN)

ANOTHER HOUR OF SLEEP.

YOU EARNED THAT SHIT!

NOTEWORTHY SHIT

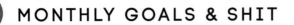

MONTHLY GOALS & SHIT

FUCKING FITNESS GOALS

ANOTHER DAMN LIST

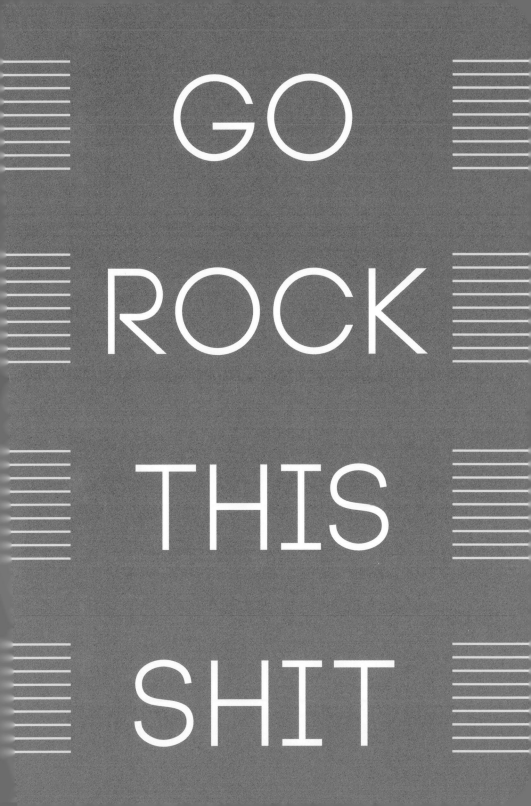

NOVEMBER

Spice That Shit Up!

2025

SUNDAY	MONDAY	TUESDAY
26	27	28
2 Daylight Saving Time ends (USA, CAN)	3	4 Election Day
9	10	11 Veterans Day (USA); Remembrance Day (CAN, UK)
16	17	18
23	24	25
30 St. Andrew's Day (SCT)		

WEDNESDAY	THURSDAY	FRIDAY	SATURDAY
29	30	31	1
5	6	7	8
12	13	14	15
19	20	21	22
26	27 Thanksgiving Day	28	29

SWEAT OUT THE BULLSHIT

DAY	ACTIVITY	TIME	DISTANCE	WEIGHT LIFTED	SETS/ REPS	

IT'S ONLY A HABIT IF YOU FUCKING DO IT.

HABIT	M	T	W	TH	F	SA	SU
Drink enough water, bitch.							

NOVEMBER

MONDAY 》
3

TUESDAY 》

Election Day

4

GET OFF YOUR ASS AND VOTE!

WEDNESDAY 》
5

THURSDAY 》
6

FRIDAY 》
7

SATURDAY 》
8

SUNDAY 》
9

NOTEWORTHY SHIT

SWEAT OUT THE BULLSHIT

DAY	ACTIVITY	TIME	DISTANCE	WEIGHT LIFTED	SETS/ REPS	

IT'S ONLY A HABIT IF YOU FUCKING DO IT.

HABIT	M	T	W	TH	F	SA	SU
Drink enough water, bitch.							

NOVEMBER

MONDAY ≫
10

TUESDAY ≫
11

Veterans Day (USA);
Remembrance Day (CAN, UK)

WEDNESDAY ≫
12

THURSDAY ≫
13

FRIDAY ≫
14

SATURDAY ≫
15

SUNDAY ≫
16

NOTEWORTHY SHIT

SWEAT OUT THE BULLSHIT

DAY	ACTIVITY	TIME	DISTANCE	WEIGHT LIFTED	SETS/ REPS	

IT'S ONLY A HABIT IF YOU FUCKING DO IT.

HABIT	M	T	W	TH	F	SA	SU
Drink enough water, bitch.							

NOVEMBER

MONDAY »
17

TUESDAY »
18

WEDNESDAY »
19

THURSDAY »
20

FRIDAY »
21

SATURDAY »
22

SUNDAY »
23

NOTEWORTHY SHIT

SWEAT OUT THE BULLSHIT

DAY	ACTIVITY	TIME	DISTANCE	WEIGHT LIFTED	SETS/ REPS	

IT'S ONLY A HABIT IF YOU FUCKING DO IT.

HABIT	M	T	W	TH	F	SA	SU
Drink enough water, bitch.							

NOVEMBER

MONDAY »
24

TUESDAY »
25

WEDNESDAY »
26

THURSDAY »
27

Thanksgiving Day

THANK-FULLLLLLL AS FUCK.

FRIDAY »
28

SATURDAY »
29

SUNDAY »
30

St. Andrew's Day (SCT)

HOW THE HELL ARE
THERE STILL LEFTOVERS?

NOTEWORTHY SHIT

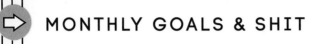

MONTHLY GOALS & SHIT

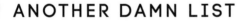

FUCKING FITNESS GOALS

ANOTHER DAMN LIST

FINISH

FUCKING

STRONG

DECEMBER

20 25

SUNDAY	MONDAY	TUESDAY
30	1	2
7 Pearl Harbor Day	8	9
14 Hanukkah begins	15	16
21 Winter begins (Northern Hemisphere)	22	23
28	29	30

WEDNESDAY	THURSDAY	FRIDAY	SATURDAY
3	4	5	6
10	11	12	13
17	18	19	20
24 Christmas Eve	25 Christmas Day	26 Kwanzaa begins; Boxing Day (AUS, CAN, NZ, UK)	27
31 New Year's Eve	1	2	3

SWEAT OUT THE BULLSHIT

DAY	ACTIVITY	TIME	DISTANCE	WEIGHT LIFTED	SETS/ REPS	

IT'S ONLY A HABIT IF YOU FUCKING DO IT.

HABIT	M	T	W	TH	F	SA	SU
Drink enough water, bitch.							

DECEMBER

MONDAY
1

CAFFEINATE AND FUCKING DOMINATE.

TUESDAY
2

WEDNESDAY
3

THURSDAY
4

FRIDAY
5

SATURDAY
6

SUNDAY
7

Pearl Harbor Day

NOTEWORTHY SHIT

SWEAT OUT THE BULLSHIT

DAY	ACTIVITY	TIME	DISTANCE	WEIGHT LIFTED	SETS/ REPS	

IT'S ONLY A HABIT IF YOU FUCKING DO IT.

HABIT	M	T	W	TH	F	SA	SU
Drink enough water, bitch.							

DECEMBER

MONDAY »
8

TUESDAY »
9

WEDNESDAY »
10

THURSDAY »
11

FRIDAY »
12

SATURDAY »
13

SUNDAY »   Hanukkah begins
14

THAT'S HOW I FUCKING ROLL.

NOTEWORTHY SHIT

SWEAT OUT THE BULLSHIT

DAY	ACTIVITY	TIME	DISTANCE	WEIGHT LIFTED	SETS/ REPS	

IT'S ONLY A HABIT IF YOU FUCKING DO IT.

HABIT	M	T	W	TH	F	SA	SU
Drink enough water, bitch.							

DECEMBER

MONDAY »
15

TUESDAY »
16

WEDNESDAY »
17

THURSDAY »
18

FRIDAY »
19

SATURDAY »
20

SUNDAY »
21
Winter begins
(Northern Hemisphere)

BABY, IT'S COLD AS SHIT OUTSIDE.

NOTEWORTHY SHIT

SWEAT OUT THE BULLSHIT

DAY	ACTIVITY	TIME	DISTANCE	WEIGHT LIFTED	SETS/ REPS	

IT'S ONLY A HABIT IF YOU FUCKING DO IT.

HABIT	M	T	W	TH	F	SA	SU
Drink enough water, bitch.							

DECEMBER

MONDAY

22

TUESDAY

23

Christmas Eve

WEDNESDAY

24

Christmas Day

THURSDAY

25

MERRY CHRISTMAS, YA FUCKING FILTHY ANIMALS!

Kwanzaa begins;
Boxing Day (AUS, CAN, NZ, UK)

FRIDAY

26

SATURDAY

27

SUNDAY

28

NOTEWORTHY SHIT

SWEAT OUT THE BULLSHIT

DAY	ACTIVITY	TIME	DISTANCE	WEIGHT LIFTED	SETS/ REPS	

IT'S ONLY A HABIT IF YOU FUCKING DO IT.

HABIT	M	T	W	TH	F	SA	SU
Drink enough water, bitch.							

DECEMBER/JANUARY

MONDAY »
29

TUESDAY »
30

WEDNESDAY »   New Year's Eve
31

CONGRATS! DO IT ALL AGAIN NEXT FUCKING YEAR.

THURSDAY »   New Year's Day
1

FRIDAY »   Day after New Year's Day (NZ, SCT)
2

SATURDAY » | **SUNDAY** »
3 | 4

NOTEWORTHY SHIT

MORE CALENDARS & GIFTS TO SWEAR BY

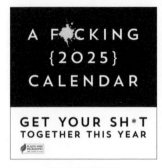

WALL CALENDAR

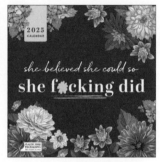

WALL CALENDAR

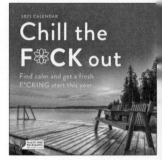

WALL CALENDAR

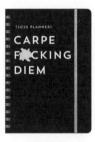

PLANNER

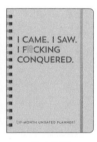

PLANNER

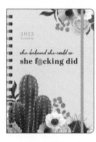

PLANNER

BOXED CALENDAR

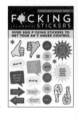

STICKERS

Copyright © 2024 by Sourcebooks
Cover and internal design © 2024 by Sourcebooks
Cover and internal design by Jillian Rahn/Sourcebooks
Cover images © sv_sunny/Getty Images
Internal images © liz Borchert/Noun Project, Maxim Filitov/Getty Images, Mooms/Noun Project, panuwach/Freepik, platypusmi86/Freepik, prettywoman/Getty Images, rastudio/Freepik, RLT_Images/Getty Images, shuoshu/Getty Images, ssstocker/Freepik, Sudowoodo/Getty Images, sv_sunny/Getty Images, user9023173/Freepik, user15245033/Freepik, varfa/Freepik

Jewish and Muslim holidays begin at sundown.

Published by Sourcebooks
P.O. Box 4410, Naperville, Illinois 60567-4410
(630) 961-3900
sourcebooks.com

Printed and bound in China.
OGP 10 9 8 7 6 5 4 3 2 1